Rev Up Your Recruiting

Acknowledgments

Any time that you have a goal to do something and you actually accomplish that goal, there will be a group of people that helped you along the way and I have to thank the wonderful mentors that I have had that made it possible. To my first mentor, Susan Orr, I send up a heavenly thank you! You taught me to believe in myself and because of that, I have never thought anything was impossible. You told me over and over again that I can do anything I want if I just work for it, and you know what? You're right. All it takes is one person to change a life and you positively changed mine when you became my baton coach, then my mentor and then my friend.

To Tawnie Cortez and Susan Hammerstrom, you are two amazing women! You came into my life when my career was just starting. What you taught me about business, customer relationships and career success is invaluable. I cannot thank you enough for the time and energy that you invested in helping me be successful.

To my kids, Garrett and Gavin, thank you for believing in me. When I left my job and said that I was going to write a book, you had no doubts about whether I would do it. You just thought it would be "chill," so thank you for believing in me. I hope that I have made you proud. And to my family, I love all of you so much!

The History of This Book

When I first started my career in college admissions, we learned a consultative sales process that helped us to learn about our students, share information about the college and determine if the college would be a good fit for them. This 4-step process was integral in helping thousands of students start their educational careers. As a new admissions representative and a new college grad, I was hesitant about being too "salesy" and about people saying no when I asked them to enroll. What I found out through time and practice is that this was much more about finding the right fit for potential students. Did our college want to have potential students enroll? Yes, of course, but we wanted students to enroll who were going to learn skills that would help them achieve their academic and career goals and we wanted students who would graduate. If I could do my part in helping them discover if college was a good fit, I could change lives and make a huge impact! As I mastered this process, I realized that consistency was the key to success and if I followed the process, students and their families left the school feeling heard and knowing if the school was a good fit for them.

After a few years as an Admissions Representative and recruiting hundreds of students, I was managing an admission department and had anywhere from four to forty employees in my department. Now, my role has changed from meeting with prospective students to teaching my admission representatives how to effectively complete a consultative sales process. I love teaching and training and if my team could do a great consultative sales process, our impact could be huge. We could change so many lives and we did! Our admission representative team enrolled thousands of students over a few years and our students went on to open businesses, be promoted, set a positive example for their kids and show their families that they could achieve their goals.

During this time of my career, I was blessed to have twin boys and as the boys began to grow, I knew that it was time to make a change in my career. I needed a career that allowed for more flexibility and one that allowed me to spend more time with my kids. One of my goals had always been to have my own baton twirling and dance studio. I started twirling baton when I was six years old and fell in love with the sport. I competed as a child and began teaching at sixteen years old. As my competition career began to wind down, I knew I wanted to twirl in college and was lucky enough to earn a coveted spot at the University of Arizona. As a twirler at the University of Arizona, I continued to teach and knew that someday I wanted to have a studio of my own.

While working in higher education that dream was still there just waiting for the right time and having busy preschoolers was the perfect opportunity to start this new adventure. I opened my baton twirling and dance studio in 2002. When I opened my business, I had just 14 students and knew that with rent and other bills, I would need to grow this business fast to make ends meet. How could I connect with families and have them choose our studio when there were four other studios in our market that were all amazing? I knew that my one secret weapon was my consultative sales process. I knew how to connect with families, learn about what they wanted and needed, and see if we were going to be the best fit for them. I implemented the consultative sales process adapted to work for a dance and baton studio. I'll share with you how to adapt it too! I loved consultative sales for getting to know parents and families, connecting on a deeper level and making sure that we were the best fit for their child. Our studio grew from 14 students to 150 in just a couple of years. We were thriving!

One of the best things about being a small business owner is being able to adapt your business to make it work in your life and 2019 brought that moment where I knew that I needed to make a change in my business. My kids were now older, involved in sports and I was missing so much because I was teaching every night and on weekends. I wanted to be there to watch them play football, basketball and all of their sports so it was time to change our business model and move to a mobile studio model. I gave up my studio space and began renting gyms from local schools and churches. I reduced the number of classes that I offered and the number of nights that I taught. This change was a blessing as the COVID-19 pandemic hit in March 2020 and business would have been much more challenging if I had had a studio.

My next career opportunity arose when I was offered the role of preschool director at the preschool where my boys attended a few years ago. Once again, I was responsible for driving enrollment, making sure classrooms were filled and budgets were met so it was time to introduce the consultative sales process again. With a few minor adaptations, the consultative sales process was implemented again and it worked. Our classrooms were full and our preschool was doing great!

As you can see, the consultative sales process works in so many different types of businesses and industries. Keep reading and I will teach you exactly how to adapt this process for your business and your industry and with practice, you can grow your business into whatever it is that you dream it to be!

Who Will This Work For?

This recruiting process will work for many, many industries and mostly in business-to-consumer sales although the skills presented are valuable in many different professional relationships. I have seen this process implemented and make a difference in dance studios, martial arts studios, child care centers or preschools, fitness studios, gymnastics centers and cheerleading programs.

In 2023, I was mentoring a new business owner and enrollment at her dance studio was stagnant. She was averaging two to three new inquiries per week and getting no more than one enrollment per month. Rent was high, payroll was high and financial obligations were starting to really overwhelm her. She was nervous that she couldn't do this. Her confidence was shaken and she began to think that maybe she was a good dance teacher but a bad business owner. We started to chat and I was thrilled to hear that she was bringing in two to three new inquiries per week because it told me that she had people interested in her classes. In one of our conversations, we talked about what the process was once a new inquiry requested information. She quickly and confidently responded, I send them an email with a link to register! My immediate response was, "WHOA! What if you went on a date and the second that you sit down at the table for dinner, your date asks you to marry them?" We both laughed but essentially that's what she was doing to her potential new customers. Asking them to commit before they knew anything about her business or before she knew if that family was a good fit for her studio.

At that moment, I knew that we had a problem but I also knew that we could fix it! We worked through the consultative sales process and soon she had turned her stagnant enrollment into a studio that was bursting at the seams! She eventually added an additional space to her studio and kept the momentum going. Her families are happy, her retention is great and she has built a business that she can be proud of.

As of this book's publication, most of our clients are predominantly women-owned small businesses so you'll see that some of the client information that is shared leans heavily toward industries that are predominantly women-owned and operated. If you are a man and own a business, don't let this deter you. This is a process designed to help build a great business and it doesn't matter the type of business or your gender. And, if you are a male business owner who implements these techniques, reach out, we'd love your feedback and input!

Let's get some terminology squared away that we are going to use throughout the book.

Recruiting can encompass a lot of different activities, such as outreach, marketing and advertising. For the purpose of this book, we are referring to recruiting as the 4-step process that you will learn more about in the next few chapters. The term recruiting can also be used when talking about attracting employees to your business; however, we are going to focus exclusively on the recruitment of new customers or clients.

Leads or inquiries refer to the potential customers for your business that you generate through your website, ads and various other sources. Leads are people who reach out to you about your business. Leads or inquiries might reach out via a form on your website, calling your business, or meeting you or your staff at a community event.

Customers are leads that have committed to your business in some way. They have enrolled in a class or purchased something from you. Your organization or company may refer to customers as clients or students.

Metrics are the numbers that provide you with the details about how you are doing in a particular segment of your recruiting process. A textbook definition of metrics would be: Metrics are quantifiable measurements. Metrics help the business owner track progress, assess performance, and measure the success of business activities. Metrics are often operational or tactical, and provide context for business activities. They are used to identify areas of improvement, make data-driven decisions, and monitor strategies' effectiveness. Metrics are often used in financial analysis by internal managers and external stakeholders.

The metrics that we are going to focus on in this book are leads/inquiries, tours scheduled, tours attended, and enrollment. When tracking each of these metrics over time, you can have visibility into where your business is excelling and where you have opportunity to make improvements.

Another Note About Rev Up Your Recruiting

This recruiting process is not a quick fix. We are not promising that you will get 50 students or clients overnight or in the next week but rather this is a system. It's not difficult, it's practice. Remember small steps forward are better than no steps forward so try one principle per week or one principle every other week. Whatever timeline works for you, go at your own pace. There's no right or wrong pace, just always keep improving in your recruiting and you will see results.

Mastering Phone Skills

In this digital world of texts and emails, phone calls may seem to be obsolete but they still hold value. And the business owners who pick up the phone may just be the winners in the onslaught of texts and emails that our leads and customers receive. Great phone skills are a valuable skill and will help your business stand apart from the rest.

When you complete an online form, what do you expect? If you are like most of us, you are expecting an automated email or text and if you are lucky maybe an email with some personal communication. How often do you receive a phone call? It's pretty rare, in fact, I can't remember the last time I received a phone call after requesting information.

You may be thinking, "No one will answer my call!" And, while the customer may not answer, you can provide quick and valuable information to the potential customer in your voicemail. One proven strategy when a business owner calls their potential customer is to reference the email that you are going to send after that voicemail. Response rate to the email goes up over 15 percent. That's pretty good odds and makes that phone call worth the effort. Our success in converting leads into real customers is just in getting that conversation going!

For phone skills, we need to be comfortable using both the outbound and the inbound phone call. The outbound phone call is essentially cold calling. You are reaching out to a potential lead with no initiation from them. For example, a dance studio may make an outbound call to a local child care center to see if they can put marketing fliers in their lobby. You may also make an outbound phone call to an inquiry that requests more information from you.

Inbound calls are the phone calls that potential customers make to you. We love inbound calls because that customer is motivated and is taking the time to reach out to you so never let that opportunity be wasted.

Let's get into the technical information of the two types of calls.

Outbound and Inbound Sales Calls

Outbound sales and inbound sales calls are two distinct approaches to selling products or services, each with its own strategies and goals. Here's an explanation of the key differences between the two:

1. **Initiation of contact**
   - **Outbound sales:** In an outbound sales call, the salesperson initiates contact with potential customers. This typically involves cold calling, where the salesperson, director or owner reaches out to leads or prospects who may not have previously expressed interest in the product or service.
   - **Inbound sales:** In an inbound sales call, the potential customer initiates the contact by reaching out to the company first. This usually happens because the customer has shown interest in the product or service, often by filling out a contact form on the company's website, making an inquiry, or responding to marketing materials.
2. **Timing**
   - **Outbound sales:** Outbound sales calls can be made at any time, regardless of whether the customer is actively seeking a solution. Business representatives often need to convince and educate prospects about the benefits of their offering.

- **Inbound sales:** Inbound sales calls occur when the customer is already interested and may be actively seeking a solution. They are usually more receptive to the sales conversation, having taken the first step by contacting you.

3. **Customer knowledge**
   - **Outbound sales:** In outbound sales, the salesperson typically has limited information about the prospect, and the call often involves introducing the product or service from scratch. The prospect may not be familiar with the company or its offerings.
   - **Inbound sales:** In inbound sales, the customer has already shown some interest and may have gathered information about the company and its products or services. The salesperson can leverage this existing knowledge during the call.

4. **Approach and pitch**
   - **Outbound sales:** In outbound calls, salespeople need to be more persuasive and proactive. They must capture the prospect's attention quickly, identify needs, and tailor the pitch accordingly.
   - **Inbound sales:** In inbound calls, the salesperson can take a more consultative approach. They often start by understanding the customer's needs and then align the product or service to those needs.

5. **Conversion rate**
   - **Outbound sales:** Outbound sales calls typically have a lower conversion rate because they involve reaching out to a

broader audience, many of whom may not be actively looking for the offered solution.
   - **Inbound sales:** Inbound sales calls tend to have a higher conversion rate because the leads are warmer and have already expressed some level of interest.
6. **Sales cycle**
   - **Outbound sales:** The sales cycle for outbound calls is often longer, as it may require more effort to nurture and convert cold leads.
   - **Inbound sales:** Inbound sales calls usually have a shorter sales cycle because the leads are already interested and closer to making a purchase decision.

Both outbound and inbound sales calls have their place in a comprehensive sales strategy, and many companies use a combination of both approaches to maximize their sales opportunities. The choice between the two depends on the company's target audience, industry, and overall sales goals.

With an understanding of the different types of calls that you may make, it is time to dig in on how to capitalize on your phone calls to turn those leads into customers.

Using the Outbound or Cold Call to Grow Your Business

Outbound or cold calls can be a valuable way to promote your business and can often be forgotten in how busy small business owners are as they manage the many aspects of their business.

Cold calling can be a strategy for small business owners looking to expand their customer base and generate new leads. However, it can also be a daunting task if not approached strategically. Here are some essential tips to help small business owners effectively make cold calls:

1. **Prepare your pitch:** Start by crafting a concise and compelling script. Your pitch should clearly communicate your value proposition, highlighting how your product or service can solve the prospect's problem or fulfill a need. Avoid sounding scripted; aim for a natural and engaging conversation.

2. **Research your prospects:** Before making a cold call, research your potential leads. Understand their industry, pain points, and any recent news or developments related to their business. This information will help you tailor your pitch and demonstrate that you've done your homework. As a center director, dance studio owner, gym owner, you may be calling businesses that would be a business alliance for you rather than calling prospective students.

3. **Create a target list:** Rather than randomly dialing numbers, create a list of high-potential prospects. Focus on businesses or individuals that are likely to benefit from your offering. This targeted approach increases your chances of success. See the "Prospective Business Alliances" information below for additional ideas for your calls.

4. **Set clear goals:** Define your objectives for each call. Are you aiming to schedule a follow-up

meeting, gather information, or make an immediate sale? Having clear goals will help you stay focused during the conversation.

5. **Practice active listening:** When making a cold call, listen attentively to the prospect's responses. Pay attention to their needs and concerns, and adapt your pitch accordingly. Effective communication is a two-way street.

6. **Handle rejections gracefully:** Rejections are a part of cold calling. Don't take them personally. Instead, use them as opportunities to learn and improve. Ask for feedback if appropriate and thank the prospect for their time. Always think of a "no" as being one step closer to a "yes."

7. **Time your calls wisely:** Consider the best times to make your cold calls. Typically, mornings and early afternoons tend to be more receptive periods. Avoid calling during lunch breaks or late in the day when people may be rushed or less responsive.

8. **Use a CRM system:** Invest in a customer relationship management (CRM) system to track your calls, record important information about prospects, and schedule follow-up tasks. This will help you stay organized and nurture leads over time. HubSpot offers a free plan that is great when you are just getting started.

9. **Practice confidence and positivity:** Confidence is key when making cold calls. Believe in your product or service, and let your enthusiasm shine through. A positive attitude can be contagious and make prospects more receptive. Smile when you call, you can absolutely "hear" your smile on the other end of the phone.

10. **Follow up consistently:** Don't expect immediate results from a single call. Follow up with prospects regularly but not too frequently. Building a relationship may take time, and persistence often pays off.
11. **Seek training and feedback:** Follow people on social media who specialize in sales. They can provide you with great tips and tricks for improving your skills. Additionally, gather feedback from colleagues or mentors to identify areas where you can enhance your approach.
12. **Comply with regulations:** Familiarize yourself with telemarketing and cold calling regulations in your area. Ensure that you're in compliance with laws regarding unsolicited calls and data protection.
13. **Track and analyze results:** Keep records of your calls and outcomes. Analyze your results regularly to identify patterns, refine your approach, and measure your return on investment (ROI).
14. **Stay persistent and patient:** Cold calling can be challenging, and success may not come overnight. Stay persistent and remember that building relationships and trust takes time.

15. **Offer a gift or bonus:** Business owners are busy and handling many tasks and responsibilities so provide your potential alliance a small gift. This can be a nice touch to show that you care and are interested in a long-term relationship. Here are a few ideas for gifts. Buy gift bags from your local dollar store and fill it with small items. You could do a self care bag with lotion, bath bombs and masks. You could do an office supply bag with colorful pens, post-it notes, motivational stickers. All these

things can be purchased online through Amazon in bulk. You can also drop these off at your local businesses and develop a relationship in person instead of starting with a phone call.

Cold calling can be an effective strategy for small business owners to generate leads and grow their customer base. By preparing thoroughly, targeting the right prospects, and consistently refining your approach, you can increase your chances of success and turn cold calls into valuable opportunities for your business.

Create a Plan for Your Outbound or Business Alliance Calls

We have curated a list of potential businesses for you to reach out to in your area. A business alliance is a formal or informal partnership with a business that serves the same customers as you do. For example, as a dance studio owner, you may partner with a tutoring center to offer a discount to the customer base of the tutoring center. In turn, the tutoring center may offer a discount to your customers.

First, decide how much time you will dedicate to growing your business through alliances per week. Will you dedicate one day per week? Will you dedicate 2 hours per week? For this example, let's say that you will be dedicating 2 hours per week to work on your business alliances.

The second step is to decide which type of business to focus on this week. For this example, the dance studio owner is going to focus on child care centers. Our dance studio owner is going to reach out to all of the child care centers within a 10 mile radius of her studio.

Here is a list of potential businesses for you to create an alliance with:

Dance studios

Gymnastics centers

Yoga studios

Tutoring centers, e.g., Sylvan Learning Center

Child care centers

Preschools

Indoor playgrounds

Indoor fun centers

Martial arts studios

Pediatric dental office

Pediatric doctor office

Make a list of businesses that you could contact to develop a relationship or alliance.

Now that you have created a plan for how often you are going to work on your business alliances and what your focus is for that week, it is time to start practicing your phone skills. The skills below provide you with the framework for calling potential business alliances. Confidence comes from practice so take the time to practice these skills and scripts alone and with a friend or family member who will role-play with you. It will feel silly but the practice helps you to develop a natural and confident conversation.

Building Confidence in Your Calls

Speaking confidently on a sales phone call is crucial for building trust with potential customers. Confidence can be the difference between success and failure in relationship building and sales. Here are some key tips to help you speak confidently on a sales phone call:

1. Preparation is key: Before the call, research the prospect, understand their needs, and know your product or service inside out. Having a clear understanding of what you're offering and who you're speaking to will boost your confidence. Let's use our example of the dance studio owner building an alliance with child care center directors. What does the Child Care Center Director need? What do they struggle with? What can you as a dance studio owner offer them? You could start with

exchanging fliers that promote each of your businesses.

Now, let's try to elevate that relationship with a partnership where your dance teacher comes to the child care center to teach a class. Each child that participates in the class receives a small gift and flier from the dance studio owner.

Or, the child care center director brings students to your studio for a gross motor play time during the winter when it is cold outside and kids need to play and move.

Could the dance studio owner offer an open gym or play time to the customers of the child care center?

As you build your relationship with your business alliance partners, you can create amazing experiences for your customers.

2. Positive mindset: Start with a positive mindset. Believe in the value of your product or service and the benefits it can bring to the customer. Confidence often stems from a strong belief in what you're selling.

3. Speak clearly and slowly: Enunciate your words clearly and maintain a steady, moderate pace.

Avoid speaking too quickly, as it can make you sound nervous or unprofessional.

When you first start calling potential business alliances, it is so easy to rush through your call and verbally "explode" on your potential customer. Take a deep breath and share all the great ideas that you have to help both of you grow your business.

4. Active listening: Show that you're engaged and genuinely interested in the prospect's needs. This not only builds rapport but also helps you tailor your pitch to their specific requirements.

   As you talk with your potential business alliances, ask questions about what struggles they are facing in their business? Are leads and inquiries hard to come by? Are they struggling with enrollment or retention? No matter the industry, all of us tend to struggle with an area of our business. Ask questions and share how your business might be able to help with their challenge.

5. Confidence in your tone: Project confidence through your tone of voice. Avoid a monotone delivery and infuse enthusiasm into your speech. Smiling while you speak can also make your voice sound more confident and friendly.

6. Practice: Rehearse your sales pitch and common objections with a colleague or in front of a mirror. Practice will help you become more comfortable with the material and reduce anxiety.

7. Handle objections gracefully: Anticipate objections and have well-prepared responses. Respond calmly and confidently, addressing the prospect's concerns while highlighting the value of your offering.

8. Use powerful words: Choose your words carefully. Use strong, persuasive language that emphasizes the benefits of your product or service. Phrases like "improve confidence" or "grow in their independence" can instill confidence in your pitch. Avoid minimizers! Minimizers are words that bring down the importance of what you do. Phrases like, "I think …" or "Tell me a little about …"

9. Ask open-ended questions: Encourage conversation by asking open-ended questions that require more than a simple yes or no answer. This engages the prospect and shows that you're interested in their perspective.

10. Handle rejection positively: Not every call will end in a sale. Accept rejection gracefully and view it as an opportunity to learn and improve. Maintain your confidence even in the face of rejection, as it's a part of the sales process.

11. Take breaks: If you have a long day of sales calls, take short breaks in between to recharge. Confidence can wane when you're tired or stressed, so stepping away for a few minutes can help you regain your composure. Set a goal and do a few calls per day.

12. Record and review calls: Record your sales calls and listen to them later. This allows you to analyze your performance objectively, identify areas for improvement, and refine your approach. Avoid words or phrases such as "well" or "um."

13. Seek feedback: Ask for feedback from colleagues or supervisors. Constructive criticism can help you fine-tune your sales pitch and boost your confidence.

14. Continual learning: Stay up to date on sales techniques and industry trends. The more knowledge you have, the more confident you'll be when discussing your product or service.

15. Visualize success: Before making the call, take a moment and visualize a successful outcome. Imagine the prospect being enthusiastic about your offering and closing the deal. Positive visualization can help boost your confidence.

16. Hit the pavement. If you are looking to try a different approach than calling or emailing businesses, try visiting your potential business alliances at their location. Bring a small gift or gift basket along with information about your business. Share with the person at the desk or the business owner (if you are lucky enough to catch them) about you, your business and that you are hoping to partner to grow both of your businesses.

In conclusion, speaking confidently on a sales phone call requires thorough preparation, a positive mindset, effective communication skills, and continuous improvement. By following these tips, you can build your confidence and increase your chances of success in sales calls. Remember, confidence is a skill that can be developed with practice and determination.

Voicemail Phone Script for Outbound or Business Alliance Phone Calls

You have developed your plan, your pitch and you are ready to get started on this new way to grow your business. Here are a few examples of scripts that you can use. Be sure to practice each script and change the wording to sound natural to you.

Hello! This message is for (Insert name of manager or owner)*. This is (Insert your name) at (Insert your business name). I am wondering if you would be interested in a partnership to promote each other's businesses to our customer base? I'd love to visit with you about several options that I have thought of on how a relationship could benefit both of us. You can call me at 555-555-5555. Looking forward to talking with you!

Phone Script for Business Alliances

Hello! This is (Insert your name) calling from (Insert your business name). I am wondering if it makes sense for us to have a conversation about a relationship that could help build both of our businesses?

Potential customer: Sure—I have a few minutes.

You: Great! Our business serves children ages three to five providing preschool education for over twenty years and I am wondering if we could put fliers at your location to promote our preschool program? The fliers would offer your families a bonus* for enrolling at our preschool. In turn, we could put a flier for your business in our entryway and put your logo and description of your business in our weekly newsletter.

Potential customer: Sounds great to me! How should we get this started?

Phone Script for Business Alliances

Hello! This is (Insert your name) calling from (Insert your business name). I am wondering if it makes sense for us to have a conversation about a relationship that could help build both of our businesses?

Potential customer: Sorry—I'm busy and don't have time.

You: OK—no problem! I've got a gift basket for you and your employees that I'm going to drop off this week. I'll throw information in there about my business and a few options that we might have for partnering. Would it make sense for me to follow up in a week?

Potential customer: Sure!

You: Super! Enjoy the basket and I'll chat with you in a week.

Potential customer: Thank you. Bye.

You: Bye.

Inbound Calls – These are Gold! Make the Most of Each One!

You have tackled the outbound phone call, which most salespeople will tell you is the most difficult of the two sales calls, so now let's move on to the inbound sales call. These are great calls because the customer is contacting you so they are motivated and seeking information! They are actively interested in learning more about your business and are reaching out to you so make the most of every call. The goal of the inbound phone call is not just to answer their questions; rather, your number one goal is to start building a relationship and (if applicable) set up a tour. Setting up a tour should be the goal for any business that has a physical location for leads to visit. In the next step of the recruiting process, you are going to learn and refine your interview skills on the tour. Here are sample questions you should ask in your phone call with your leads.

Questions to Ask In an Outbound or Inbound Call

Tell me about your child. Are they shy or outgoing?

What is their age?

What are you looking for in a dance school, preschool, gymnastic class?

Has your child been to dance, preschool or gymnastics?

When are you looking to start?

Once you have general information that allows you to know that this family could be a good fit for your business then you are going to recommend that they take a tour. Here's a transition statement that allows you to move from asking questions to directing what needs to happen next.

"It sounds like Timothy would be a great fit here. What I recommend is that we set up a time to meet so that you can see our facility, meet our teachers and I can get you all the information that you need. Are you available today at 2 pm or tomorrow at 10 am?"

If no tour, do you have a couple of minutes and I could go over the information from the tour with you? Follow the new lead interview.

Voicemail Phone Script for Leads

Hello, (Insert parent name). This is (Insert your name) from (Insert your business name). You had requested some information from us and I wanted to connect with you to give you that information. Give me a call at 555-555-5555. I'm also going to send you an email, feel free to reply to that email as well. Look forward to talking with you!

Phone Script for Outbound Call to New Lead

You: Hello! Is Sue there?

Parent: Yes—this is Sue.

You: Sue, this is (Insert your name) from (Insert your business). You requested information about our business and I'm just calling you to give you that information.

Parent: OK.

You: Sue, you mentioned in your email that you are looking for dance classes for your four-year-old. Is that correct?

Parent: Yes

You: Tell me about your child (if you can use the child's name, do so).

Parent: She's busy and loves to pretend to be a ballerina so we're just looking at dance classes for her.

You: We have a lot of students who love to be ballerinas. When are you looking to start classes?

Parent: Soon or whenever you have available.

You: Perfect! We have a class available starting next week. Would you like to come and take a tour?

Parent: Sure.

You: Wonderful! We could meet tomorrow at 4 p.m. or 7 p.m., which works best for you?

Parent: 4 pm would be great

You: Excellent! I'm going to send you an email with directions to our studio so be on the look-out for that email.

Here's a pro tip: Choose a day that is close to the date that the lead is calling. People have more motivation when it happens near the time they take action and give them two options for taking a tour. You don't want to tell them to choose a time because you are wide open … First, that communicates that you are not busy and you are—even if you are building your business. Second, people struggle with choosing when there are too many options so offering them "4 p.m. or 7 p.m." allows them to tell you if that works or offer up an alternative day and time if it doesn't work for them.

At this point, you have learned about how to make effective phone calls for both incoming and outgoing calls along with business development calls and maybe you are still skeptical about whether this will actually work for you. Here are a few examples and I want you to think about if you were the customer.

In the first example, you are calling my small business to sign up for a coach's seminar. In this example, you call at 8 p.m. and I am busy teaching so you leave a voicemail with your name and phone number. The next day, I call you back and also leave a message that says, *"Thank you for calling. I am excited to have you attend the coach's seminar. You can go to our website at bestwebsite.com/coach and sign up there."* There's nothing wrong with this approach but does it do anything to make you excited or feel appreciated? Nope.

Now think about if you leave that same message and I return your phone call and say, *"Hello, Lindsay, thank you for calling and I am really excited to have you join us for the coach's seminar. I'm going to give you a call back this evening because I am really looking forward to hearing about what part of the coach's seminar you are most interested in and what topics are the most important to you. I can also help get you registered over the phone. My number is 612-555-1212 and I am available throughout today and I'll try you again tonight around 7 p.m."*

What's your impression of my business now? In just one short voicemail, I have conveyed to you that I am excited to have you join us, interested in what information you are looking to learn and am here to help you get registered. As the customer, if you were choosing between two different businesses for a seminar and one business left you the first voicemail and one left you the second voicemail, who would you choose to give your money to?

Here's another example: You complete a form on my website to learn more about my coach's seminar. In example one, you receive this email:

Hi Lindsay, thank you for your interest in our seminar. You can sign up at <u>bestwebsite.com/coach</u> and if you have any questions, please reach out at any time.

Look forward to seeing you at the conference.

Jacinda

Again, there's nothing wrong with this email. It's friendly and provides the information that you want to know but let's try to level this up and see how we feel about the business.

Once you receive the form on the website, you call your potential customer and follow up with an email.

When you call, Lindsay doesn't answer so you leave this message:

"Hello, Lindsay, thank you for filling out our online form. I am really excited to learn more about what topics interest you the most in the coach's seminar and answer any questions that you may have. I am going to send you an email as well so feel free to call me back at 612-555-1212 or you can reply to my email. Look forward to chatting with you!"

Right after this voicemail, hit send on this email:

Hi Lindsay, thank you for your interest in our coach's seminar! We are really excited about the speakers that we have coming and what we are going to learn that day. I would love to chat with you about what questions you may have and what topics you would like to learn more about during our seminar. I have also included a link to a bio on each of our presenters below.

Feel free to send an email with any questions you may have!

I look forward to talking with you!

Jacinda

(Be sure to include links in your email)

If you are choosing between two businesses and one calls and sends an email and one sends an automated or even a nonautomated email but with no personalization, almost everyone is going to choose the more personal touch. Now, if you own any business that serves families and they are leaving their children with you, think about which business you trust more with your child. The one where you have heard the voice of the owner or voice of an employee? Or the one that sends you a short email? Most people are going to choose the business that took a little more time to assist them because you are starting to build a trustworthy relationship.

Effective phone skills are critical to improving your recruiting strategy and now we want to monitor your success. The goal of monitoring your success is not to feel bad about what you have or haven't done in the past but to find out your baseline information. This information is called metrics and can give you insight into what is going well for your business and what needs more attention, learning or training. For the week or two that you are learning and practicing these techniques, monitor your phone call metrics.

How many incoming leads do you have in a week? Define your week: Do you want to start on Sunday at 12:00 a.m. and end on Saturday at 11:59 p.m.? Be consistent with how you measure and monitor your metrics so that you are as close as possible to the same parameters each week.

Or, would you like to run your metrics on Fridays before the weekend? If so, define your week as Friday 8 a.m. to Friday 7:59 p.m.

Once you have defined what your week is going to be then measure the following things:

How many new leads do you receive in a week?

How many of those new leads did you have personal contact with this week?

Did you email and/or call each of your new leads?

How many of those leads set up a tour?

How many of those leads are enrolled in your classes?

Now that you have learned about effective phone call strategies, implement these techniques and monitor your metrics. What are your metrics when you begin this process? What are your metrics after two weeks of implementing these new skills? What are your metrics after four weeks of implementing these new skills? Are you seeing stability, growth or decline? Whatever you are seeing in your conversions helps you to know what area of your recruiting process to focus on improving.

Now that you are mastering effective phone skills, you are going to focus on the tour or the interview that you conduct with your new leads. Your tours or interviews are an integral part of developing relationships that lead to more enrollments and long-term customers.

Consider all five senses when scheduling a tour for prospective families. Here are some prompts for ensuring that your space appeals to prospective families:

Is your space clean and tidy?

Is the garbage empty or overflowing?

Are classroom supplies put away?

Does it look organized?

Is it well lit? Can you add lights to corners?

Does your space smell good? Could you have a diffuser to provide a subtle scent that appeals to families?

What is on your walls? Motivational posters? Pictures of students?

Do you play soft music in the background?

If you are unsure of how others perceive your space, ask a friend or family member who will give you honest feedback about their perception. Or, ask current families what their impression was when they visited your space for the first time.

Make adjustments as necessary to make a positive impression on prospective families. Here is a short article on why appearances are important:

https://www.retailcustomerexperience.com/blogs/the-real-impact-of-store-appearance-on-your-bottom-line/

Now that you have a family coming to visit you in person, it is time to connect and sell your services to them! In the next pages, we will explore the in-person tour and how this is the next step to increasing your enrollment.

Once your space is appealing to prospective families, now it is time to connect with your families! You are going to learn about a 3-step interview process that is critical in the recruitment process. Step 1 is to learn about the prospective family through asking thorough questions. Step 2 is to share about your organization. Step 3 is to share how the prospective family can enroll and start with your business.

Step 1 – Welcome, Introductions & Questions

Welcome your prospective family to your facility. In your welcome, include a brief introduction of yourself and then provide a brief overview of what their tour or time with you will cover. This allows you to take control of the conversation and prevents the customer from "rapid-firing" questions at you.

Here is an example of a Welcome & Introductions:

"Hello, Melissa. Thank you for coming to visit our studio. My name is Jacinda and I'm the director here. Today, we're going to take a look at our facility, talk about what you are looking for in classes and see if we are a fit for you."

<u>Why does this work?</u> First, we used the prospective customer's name. Everyone loves to hear their name so we have connected on a basic level. Second, you have described who you are and established that you are an expert for this business. You have also kept it very brief about yourself, which allows the focus to be on the parent. Third, you have established an agenda for their time with you. Typically, parents will want to know about how much it will cost and what the time commitment is. You have stated that you are going to cover that with them so that parents can focus on all of the other things that you are going to share with them. Lastly, you have taken away the pressure of "selling" or from the parent's perspective of "being sold to" by stating that you are trying to see if this is a fit for the parent and a fit for you.

Once your introductions are complete then you can begin with your questions. Here are sample questions that work across a wide variety of industries and what these questions are trying to identify.

Tell me about your child.

Parents love to talk about their kids and share about what an amazing person their child is for your business.

What is their age?

This helps you to identify what class this child will be in when they enroll.

What is their personality like?

This allows you to get to know the child and what they may need to successfully transition into your business. If they are shy, you might need to help parents know how to transition the child into the class. If they are outgoing, you may need to assist with introducing them to their new classmates.

Have they ever been in a preschool/dance/gymnastics/martial arts class before?

This helps you to identify if the child will separate easily or if that might be a challenge. This might also help you gauge a parent's experience and comfort level with leaving their child.

What did they love about the class? What did they dislike?

This is helping you identify what the child and the parents liked/disliked about their previous class/school. You can then highlight these things on your tour or this may be a talking point in your conversation about what you offer and how that differs from their previous experience.

What did you like about the preschool/dance studio/gymnastics center?

This is helping you identify what they liked or disliked about their previous experience. If they share with you that they have not attended anywhere previously then skip this question.

What are your goals for your child when they attend here?

With this question, you are identifying what parents are looking for in a visit to your facility. Be sure to ask follow-up questions that help you truly understand what parents are seeking.

When would you like your child to start with us?

Now, you are starting to identify information so that you can begin to make a class or program recommendation.

What type of schedule works best for you?

You are starting to identify any objections or obstacles that parents may have to enrolling in your program or business. If parents state they are only interested in a full-time preschool and you only offer a part-time schedule then you can begin to develop solutions for them.

Are there any things that worry you about registering and beginning class with us?

This has the parent identify if there are any potential obstacles that may stop them from enrolling with you so that you have the opportunity to discuss them before you ask them to register.

Close Out Step 1. Transition Question.

At the end of this step of the tour, you will want to ask a question that indicates to parents that you are moving on to the next step. Here are several examples of transition questions:

If I answer your questions about tuition, schedule and teacher qualifications, are there any other questions that I can answer for you?

Do you have any questions or concerns that I can address as we tour the facility?

Interview Questions – Reword these so that they are in your own words. Add additional questions that are needed for your specific program.

Tell me about your child.

What is their age?

What is their personality like?

Have they ever been in a preschool/dance/gymnastics/martial arts class before?

What did they love about the class?

What did they dislike?

What did you like about the preschool/dance studio/gymnastics center?

What are your goals for your child when they attend here?

When would you like your child to start with us?

What type of schedule works best for you?

Are there any things that worry you about registering and beginning class with us?

Is there anything else that you would like to share about your child?

Are you looking at any other preschools/dance studios/cheer studios?

If I answer your questions about tuition, schedule and teacher qualifications, are there any other questions that I can answer for you?

Step 2 – Tour & Information About Your Program

Now that you have spent time learning about your prospective family, you can begin to share more about your program. Develop and practice your speech or pitch about your business or facility. Below are two examples. The first is for a dance studio and the second is for a preschool.

First, provide a short transition statement that informs parents that you are going to transition from learning about them to sharing about your program.

An example is below:

"Let's go take a look at our school and talk about what our school has that you might enjoy."

"Let's take a look at our studio and I'll show you some of the things that make us great."

Write your own transition statement:

Now, provide information about your school, your values, the events and what it is like to be a member of your school, studio or community. A visual representation is always a nice addition to have to complement your speech or pitch. This could be a hand-out, bulletin board or video.

Here is an example for a dance studio:

Our studio has four core values that we try to weave into each class. These values are confidence, leadership, friendship and growth.

We build children's confidence by encouraging each student to reach their potential with positive language and positive affirmations. We want them to improve in comparison to where they are without comparing themselves to others. We accomplish this with small class sizes of ten or less so that their teacher can connect with them.

If we take a look over here, you'll see our classroom leaders. We encourage all of our students to be a leader in their classroom starting with our youngest classes. We know that our students use those leadership skills in high school, college and beyond and we begin leadership training on their first day. Our teachers do annual training on leadership and mentoring our next generation of leaders through high standards, discipline and compassion.

Now, if you take a look at our Facebook page or this bulletin board, you'll see that we want students to connect and grow their friendships with their classmates. These friendships often last well into adulthood so we run a "sister" program along with events that help deepen those bonds. Families love our annual banquet, our annual recital, bowling with their team and studio sleepover.

One thing that we focus on in every class is continuous growth. This growth is important for improvement, but also for learning to be resilient and have grit. We know that students will face challenges but we work with them on how they can work toward continuing to practice, learn and grow.

Does this sound like the right environment for your child? Does this sound like it is a match for your family's values?

This question is important in closing out Step 2 and identifying if your prospective family has any objections and can see themself joining your school.

If they provide you with any objections or concerns, take the time to go back and explore those concerns. Ask questions to learn more about these concerns now to prevent them from walking away with the enrollment at the end of Step 3.

Create your own tour and speech here. Be sure to integrate details that are important to your families such as information about shows, recitals, costumes or other things that make your program unique. For example, if families only buy one costume, you may want to highlight that in your speech and tour.

Step 3 – Details & Registration

If your prospective family has provided you with no concerns or objections at the end of Step 1 or Step 2 then it is time to move to the details for enrolling and starting class with your business.

Create a transition statement that asks your prospective family if they have any questions or concerns before you review the enrollment and registration information.

Here is an example:

Do you have any other questions before I share our enrollment, tuition and registration information? Do we seem to be a good fit for you and your family?

Create your own transition statement:

Once you have transitioned from Step 2 into Step 3 then you will want to provide the details for your program. This is going to include things such as:

Schedule

Times

Registration fees

Tuition

And, any other expectations that parents will need to meet or know about before registering. It is important to be open, honest and up front so that parents are not surprised during the registration and beginning of classes. Here is an excellent time to provide your customers with a folder or packet of information. See the list below for ideas about what to include in your information.

Here is a sample of this information being presented to a parent:

It sounds like we are a great fit for your child and your family and we are excited to welcome you into our community. Here's what you need to do in order to get started.

I would recommend Beginner Ballet on Mondays from 5:30–6:15 for your child. You said that she loves to pretend to be a ballerina and in this class she will learn those important fundamentals of dance. Class begins on September 1 and we finish on May 1 with our annual recital.

Your class fees are $50 per month with a costume fee of $100 due in November and a recital fee of $50 due in April.

Is that what you were expecting for tuition and fees?

> This is an important question to see if you have a potential objection on cost. It is always better to face cost objections head-on and in person than to have your potential customer having doubts about their investment when they leave.

If your customer has no objection to the cost then I would move forward with registration. Explain your registration process to them. Here is an example.

Super! If that class seems like a good fit and if the tuition works with your budget then you can begin with us by completing our registration form. Once you register then your space will be held and we will send you the handbook for your review and sign-off.

Now, develop your Step 3. Think about your current process and how you are going to implement the new skills that you have just learned. Will you start from scratch or will you merge what you were doing with your new skills? What do you do well and want to keep? What do you need to remove from your process? Take time to develop questions that apply to your business and get that commitment and connection from your inquiry to your business.

Customer Packet

Parents love to have a tangible item to take with them. Create a packet or folder that includes all or a few of the things below. Add "WOW" factor by including a small gift bag for kids that includes crayons, pencils, coloring sheets or other popular toys.

Staff list & bios – Include pictures of staff and contact information. This provides parents with important information about the qualifications of your staff, how to get in touch with them and starts building that relationship.

Price list – Include tuition, any fees that you may charge, supplies that are needed. Be up front with your customers. It is always better to share this early in the process and discuss it before registration than have a parent who is upset about a surprise expense.

Important dates – Families are busy so no matter what industry you are from provide a list of dates that includes when classes begin, end, when the school is closed for holidays, performance dates, due dates for fees or forms.

Mission, vision & values – A successful organization is driven by their mission, values and vision. You can write a whole book on just this and many people have! Create a document or flier that shares what you believe and what is important to your organization. Some of this information should be shared with your customers during your tour to make sure what they need matches what you believe in and how it impacts your business. You want to make sure that parent's needs align with your business. Here's an example: I was the director at a Christian preschool. When touring with potential families, I would share about our school's beliefs and how things are done. Often parents would ask if the children pray before snack or lunch? The answer was yes, they do pray before snack and lunch. At that point, I would share how being a Christian preschool is different than a preschool that is privately owned. This information sharing was not meant to sway parents but inform about our beliefs and operations and allow parents to decide what works best for them. Most people have visited your website and have some knowledge about what your business is about but your tour is the chance to share more detail.

Registration Form (if not online)

Program explanation – Create a document that shows how students' progress through your program and the pathway(s) that they can take once they begin. For example, do students start in Beginner Ballet, proceed to

Ballet 2 and then can move to a competition track or recreational track? If you have a preschool, do students begin in the Monkey Class (three-year-old classroom) and move on to the Zebras (four-year-old classroom)?

Testimonials – Include a document or page that shares what current families are saying about your business. With permission, use real pictures of your customers and stories about their growth. Consider including an email address of a current or former customer who is willing to answer questions from incoming parents.

	Sample Week 1	Actual Week 1
New leads/inquiries	5	
Personal contact	5	
Tours scheduled	4	
Phone to scheduled tour	80% (or # of tours scheduled divided by # of new leads)	
# of tours attended	3	
Show rate conversion	75%	
# of tours enrolled	2	
Show to enrollment	66%	

conversion		
Lead to enrollment conversion	40%	

The Importance of Practice

You may be applying one or even a few of these methods right now but are nervous about adding to or changing your process. I know change is hard and it is easy to return to the "old way" of doing things, but you started this process because you wanted to improve your business and these techniques will improve your business. I have used this process for over twenty years and it can work in a variety of industries so be patient with yourself as you develop and implement these changes. You can do this!

Now, take a few minutes and decide on your strategy for implementation. Are you adding your new phone skills and the interview at once? Are you doing new phone skills for three weeks and then the interview techniques? Choose a strategy for implementation that works for you, your business and your timeline. Write your strategy down and put it in a prominent spot. Work on this new style of recruiting as much as you need to for it to be comfortable. We don't promise ten new clients in a week for a reason or any other ridiculous how-to-get-rich-quick process—this is a process that takes time to become comfortable with and a slow and steady approach is just fine! You will reap the

benefits and the best part is so will your customers! You are going to build a community of people who know and love your business because you took the time to get to know them, to know their wants and needs!

Also, I cannot recommend enough the benefits of practicing your phone calls and interviews with a staff or family member. Practice will help you to feel more comfortable with asking quality questions and practicing with a staff or family member allows you to make mistakes and try different ways to say things to see what resonates with your potential customer.

Metrics

As mentioned earlier in this book, metrics are integral in helping you to measure where you are improving and what areas provide an opportunity for improvement.

Without judgment on yourself, monitor your conversions on each of these metrics.

Input the number of new leads that you have received via inbound phone calls, your website, online ads and any other ways that you are generating leads.

Personal contact is reaching out to your leads with a phone call, email or both. For a personal touch, I would reach out with both a phone call and email; however, if you do not have a phone number then reach out via email. To be honest, if you want to have an effective, customer-focused business, every new lead should have personal contact from you or a designated employee. Our businesses are built around making new leads feel appreciated and welcomed and this initial personal contact is the first step in developing a positive relationship.

Phone to scheduled tour shows you the effectiveness of your outgoing communication with your new leads. A baseline in most industries (studios, child care/preschool, tutoring centers) is 75 percent of all of your new leads should schedule a tour. Monitor this number over several weeks. If your conversion is below 75 percent then you may want to practice your phone skills to build a compelling reason for your new leads to schedule and come to a tour. Often, if we give them all of the information over the phone, they will not have a reason to come to their tour. During our phone call or email, we want to communicate a compelling reason for them to schedule and attend their tour. We want to give them enough information to pique their interest but not so much that they are overwhelmed or have all of the information they need to make a decision before visiting.

Number of tours attended – This is the number of tours that attended their scheduled time to take a tour.

Show rate conversion – This is the percentage that you will discover by dividing the number of tours that show by the number of tours that are scheduled. A show rate of 75 percent or better is standard in the studio and daycare/preschool industry.

Show to enrollment conversion – This is the percentage of people who show up for their tour that enroll. We generally see a conversion of 70 to 75 percent in this metric. This metric is showing you the effectiveness of your interview with your prospective customers. If your interview is not answering your customer's questions and you are not closing out each section of the process then you will see this number trend down. Your customers will not enroll if they have questions about your business or the process for starting with you. Pay attention to the potential customer's nonverbal cues and be brave enough to ask tough questions if you sense hesitancy. It's better to know what they are thinking now then wonder if they are ever going to come back and enroll with you.

Lead to enrollment conversion – This conversion can vary widely based on location and industry. We have seen as high as 60 percent and as low as 20 percent. Your lead to enrollment conversion is so important in how you are going to grow and maintain your business. Consider this example, you currently have twenty students but want to grow to forty students. Your business is generating four leads per week and you enroll 50 percent of those leads so you are enrolling approximately two students per week or eight students per month. You will reach your goal of forty students in two and a half months.

What impact will adding twenty students make on your business? Twenty students can change your life, your business and set you up for continued success. Small changes done over time make a big difference, so what will you do today?

Moving Forward in the Process

Imagine you have implemented the recruiting process for three months and you are tracking your metrics and seeing steady improvement; however, you are not quite where you want to be for enrollments or registrations. How can you get a little more growth? Where can you find a few more customers? The answer is the people who "fall off" during this process. The people who "fall off" during your process are easy to forget about but a vital part of this process. Continue to reach out via phone and email to these potential customers. Here are a few categories of potential customers that are waiting for you!

Inquiries

These are the people who requested information from you but never answered an email or phone call. Continue to send your inquiries information either via email or by reaching out with a phone call. Email topics could include new instructor announcements, sharing a student success story, sharing about a community event that your group will attend, promoting a special event that you will host, sharing content that your target demographic loves to consume. Phone calls could include sharing about new classes starting or sharing that you are available to answer any questions. If you have a staff member who is great on the phone, ask them to reach out on your behalf.

Inquiries That Scheduled an Appointment but Didn't Show

These people took the time to communicate with you and unfortunately did not attend their tour so they do have an interest in your business and what you offer. Continue to reach out to this group via email and phone calls. You can use the same topics for your inquiries but personalize the communication if possible. Here is an example of a short email that utilizes the information that we know about this inquiry.

Hello Sarah,

When we talked you mentioned that you were worried about Sally being able to separate from you for preschool. Here's a great blog post that has some tips and tricks for combating separation anxiety for young children. Please let me know if you have any questions on this topic! We see it quite a lot in our young students!

Insert Link Here.

Hope you are doing well!

Jacinda

This email is informative and is hopefully helping that potential customer move past an obstacle. What is great about this email is that you are not pushing enrollment, you are showing that you listened during your phone or email conversation with your potential customer and you are demonstrating that you care to help them move past an obstacle.

Inquiries That Showed for a Tour/Appointment but Did Not Enroll

The next group to focus on are the people who showed up for a tour but never enrolled. Maybe they enrolled somewhere else? But maybe they didn't and they are nervous about the time commitment or financial commitment or are just the type of person who doesn't like to finish paperwork. Those people exist!

Continue to reach out to this segment with content that would appeal to them based on your phone conversation and tours. Let them know about student successes, special events and share the content that you create that helps them to move forward with success.

These three segments of your lead base are important so continue to email and call. Provide them valuable content but personalize it to their situation. Does it take more time than blasting out a preformatted email? Yes! Will your customer know that you care and that you listened? Absolutely!

How often should you contact these potential customers? This can vary widely based on your industry, my recommendation would be to contact them weekly within a month of them requesting information about your business. Contact them biweekly starting in month two to three after they requested information and contact them monthly in months four and after.

What if they ask you to stop contacting them? If a customer shares that they have chosen to go to a different studio or they ask you to stop calling and emailing them then you need to stop reaching out to them. When they ask you to stop reaching out to them, be kind—they will remember how you treated them. Wish them the very best luck and to reach out if they ever have any questions about your industry.

Putting It All Together

If you've made it this far, you have learned about how to utilize the phone to make an impact on your business, how to connect with families during a tour or interview and how to monitor your metrics to determine your successes and areas of opportunity. If you ever find an area that decreases in effectiveness, pull this book out and revisit the basics. You will find that area rebound quickly when you return to the basic principles that make this process work.

Other Resources

If you need more small business tips, helps, follow me on

Facebook: Search batontwirlingcoach

Instagram: baton_twirling_unlimited or coachjacindamiller

Want to dive deeper? Take our self-paced, online course to learn even more about this topic:

Rev Up Your Recruiting Online Course

Jacinda's Tip #1

When you ask your potential customer and they don't answer immediately, do not rush to fill the "blank space." Get comfortable with being quiet and let your potential customer answer the question.

Jacinda's Tip #2

Don't ever say that your calendar is wide open. A better option is to give your potential customer two options for coming to visit your business. Would they like 2 p.m. on Tuesday or 7 p.m. on Wednesday?

Jacinda's Tip #3

If your customer doesn't show that does NOT mean that they are not interested. They are probably very interested in your product or service. They could be scared, nervous or forgot about their meeting with you. Call and email them to see if you can reschedule. Be kind when you call, they may also be embarrassed that they forgot or chose not to come.

Jacinda's Tip #4

No one wants to be sold to but people do like to buy. Our job is not to sell but to make sure this is a good fit for your prospective family. Work to achieve small "yes" moments with your prospective family so that they are empowered and ready to buy when you ask them.

Jacinda's Tip #5

The relationship doesn't end at closing. Follow up to ensure satisfaction, address issues, and uncover opportunities for upselling or referrals.

By focusing on the client's needs and providing tailored solutions, consultative sales representatives can build lasting relationships and achieve sustainable success.

Jacinda's Tip #6

Always ask for the enrollment or the sale! It's less work long-term for you to know where that family is in the decision-making process.

Jacinda's Tip #7

Always leave the meeting with a defined action plan. Whether it's scheduling a follow-up, providing additional materials, be clear on what comes next.

Jacinda's Tip #8

Share relatable success stories or case studies of similar clients. Show how your solution made a difference for others in their situation.